GENITAL HERPES

GENITAL HERPES

H. Hunter Handsfield

Professor of Medicine
University of Washington School of Medicine
Director, Sexually Transmitted Disease Control Program
Public Health – Seattle & King County
Seattle, Washington

McGraw-Hill

MEDICAL PUBLISHING DIVISION

New York   Chicago   San Francisco   Lisbon
London   Madrid   Mexico City   Milan   New Delhi
San Juan   Seoul   Singapore   Sydney   Toronto

McGraw-Hill

*A Division of The **McGraw·Hill** Companies*

GENITAL HERPES

1234567890   KGPKGP   09876543210

ISBN 0-07-137971-1

This book was set in Times Roman by York Graphic Services.
The editors were Martin Wonsiewicz and Scott Kurtz.
The production supervisor was Richard Ruzycka.
The cover designer was Mary McKeon.
The text designer was Marsha Cohen/Parallelogram Graphics.
The index was prepared by Alexandra Nickerson.
Figures 5–22 are reprinted from *Color Atlas and Synopsis of Sexually Transmitted Diseases, 2d ed.,* by H. Hunter Handsfield (New York: McGraw-Hill, 2001).

Quebecor World/Kingsport was printer and binder.

This book is printed on acid-free paper.

Library of Congress Cataloging in Publication Data
Handsfield, H. Hunter.
    Genital herpes/H. Hunter Handsfield.
       p.; cm.
    Includes bibliographical references and index.
    ISBN 0-07-137971-1
      1. Herpes genitalis. I. Title.
    [DNLM: 1. Herpes Genitalis. WC 578 H236g 2001]
    RC203.H45 H36 2001
    616.95'18—dc21   2001030548

CONTENTS

Except for the acquired immunodeficiency syndrome, genital herpes probably is the sexually transmitted disease of greatest concern to sexually active young adults in the United States and other industrialized countries. Questions to the Centers for Disease Control and Prevention's National STD Hotline about genital herpes greatly outnumber those about any other STDs, and all clinicians who provide STD care can testify to the frequently devastating impact of herpes for newly diagnosed patients.

To a large extent, the fears are well-founded. The prospect of lifelong carriage of a painful, recurrent, incurable, sexually transmitted infection, with potentially profound effects on current sexual relationships and the formation of new ones, is a legitimate concern. Furthermore, the increased risk of infection with human immunodeficiency virus, if exposed, is real, as is the rare but devastating occurrence of neonatal herpes. However, the truth is that most genital herpes infections are so mild that they go unnoticed by both infected persons and their doctors, and almost all cases can be controlled and complications prevented, even though cure remains elusive. It has been argued that alarmist publicity and media attention in past years contributed to the fear of herpes and to psychological morbidity in those affected, and there may be some truth to the charge. But that is a moot point; whatever their origins, clinicians must be prepared to address patients' concerns and to assuage their fears without belittling them.

It is the purpose of this short book to help clinicians achieve that goal. The *sine qua non* of excellent patient care for any clinical entity is accurate knowledge about it. Genital herpes is a complex disease, and I saw a need for a resource that filled the gap between the many excellent reviews, chapters and research papers that are available, which by definition are limited in scope, and the few available full-length books that are too long for quick reading and are written for the patient more than the clinician. I have taken a narrative approach, without specific citations; where clear documentation is lacking in the medical literature or the conclusions are contradictory, I rely on my own clinical experience and judgment. I trust that experts in herpes and other STDs will not find any outlandish statements, even if some details are debatable.

As with all books, this one relied on the help of several persons. I especially thank my colleagues, Drs. Larry Corey and Anna Wald, for their knowledge and support; most of what I know about genital herpes I learned directly or indirectly from them, and they are my touchstones for almost every aspect of the disease. Drs. Rhoda Ashley, Zane Brown, and Larry Stanberry also answered questions that arose as I wrote. Charlie Ebel read parts of the manuscript, and he and Terri Warren gave valuable advice about patient education and the psychological aspects of herpes. The American

Social Health Association, under the leadership of Linda Alexander, was a valuable resource. Finally, I thank my wife, Patricia McInturff, and my editor, Marty Wonsiewicz, for their support and assistance.

H. Hunter Handsfield
Seattle, Washington
April 14, 2001

ACV	acyclovir
AIDS	acquired immunodeficiency syndrome
CDC	Centers for Disease Control and Prevention
CMV	cytomegalovirus
DNA	deoxyribonucleic acid
EBV	Epstein-Barr virus
ELISA	enzyme-linked immunoabsorbent assay
FA	fluorescent antibody test
HHV	human herpesvirus
HIV	human immunodeficiency virus
HSV	herpes simplex virus
NHANES	National Health and Nutrition Examination Survey
PCR	polymerase chain reaction test
RPR	rapid plasma reagin
STD	sexually transmitted disease
VDRL	Venereal Disease Research Laboratory
VZV	varicella zoster virus

GENITAL HERPES

INTRODUCTION

Genital herpes is the most prevalent sexually transmitted disease (STD) in the United States; approximately 25% of the adult population is infected and up to one million persons acquire the infection annually. The term *herpes* is derived from the ancient Greek (serpent), probably in recognition of the linear, snakelike dermatomal distribution of herpes zoster. Most cases of genital herpes are caused by herpes simplex virus type 2 (HSV-2), but many infections are due to HSV type 1 (HSV-1), more commonly known as the cause of oral herpes (cold sores, fever blisters). Infection persists in neural tissue for the life of the infected person and is characterized by recurrent mucocutaneous eruptions. Most infections are subclinical; some of these are entirely asymptomatic, whereas others are characterized by nonspecific symptoms whose significance is not appreciated by infected persons and often not by clinicians. As for all inflammatory or ulcerative STDs, genital herpes enhances the efficiency of sexual transmission and acquisition of the human immunodeficiency viruses (HIV).

The incurable nature of genital herpes, the prolonged potential for transmission to sex partners even when asymptomatic, and the potential for devastating neonatal infection cause substantial psychological stress, often out of proportion to the clinical manifestations and the actual risks of serious outcomes. For these reasons, herpes is the most feared STD aside from the acquired immunodeficiency syndrome (AIDS). By contrast, many health care professionals view genital herpes as a relatively uncommon and generally trivial condition. One of the most common complaints of infected persons is that their physicians were insensitive and seemingly had little knowledge about genital herpes and its management. In fact, no other STD requires a more knowledgeable, caring, empathetic health care provider. This booklet reviews the salient features of the epidemiology, clinical manifestations, treatment, and prevention of genital herpes.

ETIOLOGY AND PATHOGENESIS

There are eight known human herpesviruses **(Table 1),** but in clinical usage the term *herpes* applies only to infections caused by HSV or varicella zoster virus. HSV is a complex, lipid-enveloped virus **(Fig. 1).** HSV-1 and HSV-2 primarily infect mucocutaneous tissues and are also neurotropic. Initial infection in adults sometimes causes acute encephalitis (HSV-1) or meningitis (HSV-2), and both viruses establish chronic infection in dorsal spinal or cranial nerve ganglia by retrograde transmission along the axons of sensory neurons. It is uncertain whether chronic neural infection is truly latent (i.e., without ongoing viral replication) or if slow replication continues during the quiescent phase. The virus intermittently migrates from the ganglia along sensory nerves, resulting in recurrent lesions of the skin or mucous membranes served by the affected neurons. It is unknown whether clinical recurrences and subclinical viral shedding result from variations in viral replication in the ganglia, from factors that influence migration down sensory axons, or from host-virus interactions at mucocutaneous surfaces; all three mechanisms may be involved.

Cellular and humoral immunity develops in response to the initial infection. Although incapable of eradicating infection, the immune response apparently prevents exogenous

Table 1. HUMAN HERPESVIRUSES

Virus	Primary Clinical Manifestations
Herpes simplex virus type 1 (HSV-1)	Mucocutaneous herpes (mostly oral, some genital)
Herpes simplex virus type 2 (HSV-2)	Genital herpes
Varicella zoster virus (VZV)	Chickenpox, herpes zoster (shingles)
Cytomegalovirus (CMV)	Mononucleosis syndrome, neonatal infections, opportunistic disease; mostly asymptomatic
Epstein-Barr virus (EBV)	Infectious mononucleosis, B-cell lymphoma, oral hairy leukoplakia; mostly asymptomatic
Human herpesvirus type 6 (HHV-6)	Roseola infantum ("Sixth disease")
Human herpesvirus type 7 (HHV-7)	Mostly asymptomatic; may mimic HHV-6
Human herpesvirus type 8 (Kaposi sarcoma herpesvirus) (HHV-8, KSHV)	Kaposi's sarcoma, B-cell lymphoma; mostly asymptomatic

reinfection with the same virus type, is responsible for resolution of the initial clinical manifestations, and results in more rapid healing of recurrent than initial outbreaks. Immunity also influences the clinical manifestations when a person who already is infected with one virus type is exposed to the other type. Specifically, when HSV-2 infection occurs in a person already infected with HSV-1, the clinical manifestations are less severe than in persons without prior HSV-1 infection. Some studies also show that HSV-1

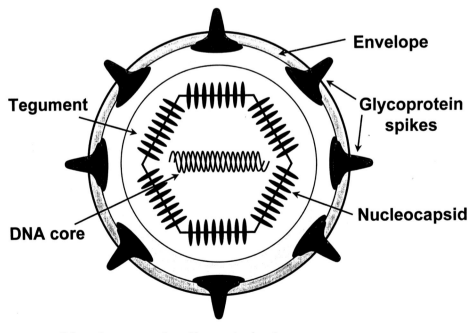

Figure 1. *Schematic representation of herpes simplex virus.*

antibody is associated with a lower risk of acquiring HSV-2 infection, in addition to reduced clinical severity, but conflicting data exist. Type-specific antibodies against the HSV surface antigen glycoprotein G1 (specific for HSV-1) or glycoprotein G2 (specific for HSV-2) are the basis of type-specific serologic tests for HSV infection.

The interactions between viral replication, immunity, and potential triggers of recrudescent infection are poorly understood. Well-established stimuli of recurrent oral HSV-1 infection include fever, intercurrent infection, and exposure to ultraviolet radiation (e.g., sunlight). Definitive triggers, however, have not been identified for recurrent genital HSV-2 infection, notwithstanding anecdotal reports and many patients' beliefs about stress, menstruation, sexual activity, diet, and other factors.

The biologic explanation for the differing anatomic tropisms of HSV-1 and -2 remains obscure. HSV-2 almost exclusively infects the genitals, anus, or surrounding areas. Oral infection with HSV-2 is uncommon except in the presence of primary genital herpes, and recurrent oral herpes is almost never due to HSV-2. By contrast, HSV-1 causes a substantial minority of genital infections. When HSV-1 causes genital infection, symptomatic recurrences and subclinical viral shedding are less frequent than in genital HSV-2 infection. Thus, type-specific antibody to HSV-2 almost always indicates sexually acquired anogenital infection, whereas HSV-1 seropositivity reflects either genital or oral infection. For these reasons, the often misused terms "herpes type 1" and "herpes type 2" are not synonymous with oral and genital herpes, respectively; the numerical designations are properly used only for the viruses, not the clinical syndromes they cause.

EPIDEMIOLOGY OF GENITAL HERPES

INCIDENCE, PREVALENCE, AND
IMPACT OF GENITAL HERPES

During the second cycle of the National Health and Nutrition Examination Survey (NHANES-II, midpoint 1978), a population-based study of health status in the United States, the seroprevalence of HSV-2 antibody was 16.7%. HSV-2 seroprevalence increased to 21.7% during NHANES-III (midpoint 1991), a 30% rise over 13 years. As shown in **Fig. 2,** the prevalence rose in all age groups, but the greatest proportionate rise, from about 2% to almost 6% prevalence, occurred in teenagers. Most persons with HSV-2 acquire the infection during the period from their teen years through to the age of 40, and HSV-2 seroprevalence is linearly related to the respondents' numbers of lifetime sex partners, as expected for an STD. By contrast, the prevalence of HSV-1 infection, most cases of which are not sexually acquired, rises in a linear fashion from early childhood through the age of 65 and is not significantly influenced by indices of sexual behavior.

Thus, in 1991 approximately 45 million persons in the United States were infected with HSV-2. Considering additional HSV-2 infections acquired during the next decade plus unknown millions of HSV-1-seropositive persons who have genital rather than oral infection, it is likely that 60 million or more persons ($>25\%$ of the adult population) have genital HSV infection. HSV-2 seroprevalence is higher in women than in men, in men who have sex with men (MSM) than in heterosexuals, and in populations with

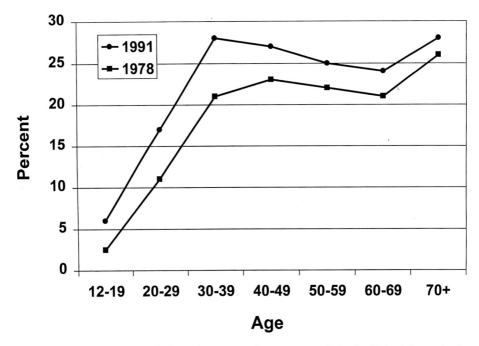

Figure 2. *Prevalence of antibody to herpes simplex virus type 2 in the United States in the National Health and Nutrition Examination Survey (NHANES) in 1976–1980 (midpoint 1988) and 1989–1994 (midpoint 1991).*

lower than high socioeconomic attainment. Not surprisingly, HSV-2 seroprevalence is higher in persons attending STD clinics than in other settings. Finally, there is substantial geographic variation, with higher prevalences of both HSV-1 and HSV-2 infection in the southeastern states and lower prevalences in the north and west.

Genital herpes is a frightening disease to sexually active young persons, out of proportion to the actual morbidity it causes. In a national, population-based, random-digit dialing telephone survey in 1999, 1,002 persons aged 18 to 40 years were read a list of potentially traumatic life events, for each of which they were asked, "How traumatic would it be for you personally: very traumatic, somewhat traumatic, not very traumatic, or not traumatic at all?" Acquiring AIDS topped the responses, rated by 96% of respondents as very traumatic. Having genital herpes was rated as very traumatic by 68% of those surveyed, substantially exceeding the proportion that classified breaking up with a significant other (54%), getting fired from a job (51%), or failing a course in school (28%) as very traumatic. **Table 2** corroborates those findings. Among 134,411 spontaneous disease-specific telephone calls to the Centers for Disease Control and Prevention's National STD Hotline in 1997, 47% of callers had questions about genital herpes, almost matching the number for all other STDs combined.

TRANSMISSION

Genital herpes in adults, whether due to HSV-1 or HSV-2, is sexually acquired. HSV-2 infection is transmitted almost entirely by genital or anal intercourse. Genital HSV-1

**Table 2. MAIN TOPICS RAISED BY CALLERS TO THE NATIONAL SEXUALLY
TRANSMITTED DISEASE TELEPHONE HOTLINE, 1997***

	No. of Calls (%)
Genital herpes	63,484 (47)
HPV/warts†	33,533 (25)
Chlamydia	17,341 (13)
Gonorrhea	11,300 (8)
Syphilis	8,753 (7)
Total	134,411

*Limited to disease-specific calls

†HPV denotes human papillomavirus.

infection evidently is transmitted both by genital intercourse and orogenital sex, but
the proportionate contribution of these two routes is unknown. Transmission probably
results from inoculation through microabrasions and is more efficient from men to
women than the reverse, probably because in women a greater surface area of moist
tissues is exposed. Consistent use of the male condom reduces transmission efficiency,
especially from men to women, but does not eliminate it.

No credible evidence supports the occurrence of HSV transmission through exposure
to infected secretions on toilet seats or by moist fomites such as bathing suits or towels.
Assertions to the contrary generally failed to recognize the possibility of acquisition from
an asymptomatic sex partner (often in a longstanding relationship) or the first occurrence
of symptoms long after subclinical initial infection. Autoinoculation of HSV from genital or oral lesions accounts for rare cases of acute herpetic keratitis, herpes whitlow, and
perhaps oropharyngeal infection. Most such infections occur in persons with initial HSV
infection, when patients should be advised to avoid manual contact with lesions and to
wash their hands before touching susceptible sites, especially the eyes. Although such
advice is also commonly given to patients with recurrent herpes, autoinoculation occurs
rarely if ever in persons with recurrent oral or genital herpes.

INTERACTIONS WITH HUMAN
IMMUNODEFICIENCY VIRUS

Genital ulcer disease and other STDs are well established as risk factors for sexual
transmission of HIV, and differences in the incidence and prevalence of STDs in the
population partly explain the wide differences in the frequency of heterosexual transmission of HIV around the world. In HIV-infected persons with herpes, HIV is present
in high concentrations in recurrent genital lesions, and case-control studies and prospective cohort studies have linked genital herpes and serologic evidence of HSV-2 infection with acquisition of HIV. In HIV-infected persons, HSV infection is associated
with increased plasma levels of HIV, perhaps adversely affecting the course of HIV
disease. The clinical course of genital herpes also is adversely affected by HIV infection, and the occurrence of chronic, debilitating mucocutaneous herpetic ulcers in persons with AIDS is well known. More recently, it has been learned that the frequency

of subclinical shedding of HSV-2 is twice as high in HIV-infected MSM with genital herpes as in those without HIV infection.

NEONATAL HERPES

An estimated 2000 to 5000 cases of neonatal herpes occur annually in the United States, with great variation around the country. The infection usually results from transmission of HSV from maternal genital infection to the infant during delivery or the perinatal period, sometimes after prolonged rupture of the fetal membranes. A few cases (probably <5%) result from postnatal exposure to a parent or caregiver with oral HSV-1 infection. The highest risk of neonatal herpes occurs when the mother first acquires genital HSV infection during the third trimester of pregnancy. In one series, neonatal herpes developed in only one infant born to 96 mothers who had asymptomatic cervical shedding of HSV at term in the presence of chronic infection, indicated by the presence of antibody to the virus type isolated. By contrast, neonatal herpes occurred in 8 (40%) of 20 infants ($P < .0001$) whose mothers had asymptomatic genital shedding of HSV-1 or HSV-2 without homologous antibody, indicating initial infection. Even when overt genital ulcers due to recurrent herpes are present at term, transmission to the newborn is uncommon, probably because maternal immunity provides substantial protection against transmission. However, because the prevalence of chronic genital herpes in pregnant women is far higher than the number who acquire HSV near term, a high proportion of neonatal herpes is attributed to recurrent maternal herpes. For these reasons, prevention of neonatal herpes depends on both preventing initial genital herpes near term and preventing neonatal exposure to recurrent herpetic lesions.

Although cesarean section continues to be recommended in the United States when pregnant women have clinically evident recurrent herpes during labor, it is likely that few cases of neonatal herpes are prevented by this strategy. Moreover, such unnecessary cesarean sections probably cause substantial maternal and neonatal morbidity, and in some countries the presence of recurrent genital herpes is no longer considered a valid indication for cesarean section. Nevertheless, in the United States medicolegal considerations dictate abdominal delivery if overt herpetic lesions are present at term. Fetal monitoring with scalp electrodes, which provides an efficient portal of entry for the virus, is also a risk factor for neonatal infection. Surveillance cultures for HSV near term are ineffective in preventing neonatal herpes and are not recommended. An alternative approach, and the subject of recent research, is to administer antiviral therapy during the last month of pregnancy to women with recurrent genital herpes. This strategy probably prevents few cases of neonatal herpes, but may avert some otherwise unnecessary cesarean sections by preventing recurrent herpes outbreaks.

CLINICAL MANIFESTATIONS OF GENITAL HERPES

CLINICAL CLASSIFICATION

As shown in **Table 3,** genital herpes can be categorized into initial infection, which is further subdivided into primary and nonprimary infection, recurrent herpes, and sub-

Table 3. CLINICAL SPECTRUM OF GENITAL HERPES

- Initial-episode infection
  —Primary infection
  —Nonprimary initial-episode infection
- Recurrent infection
- Subclinical infection
  —Asymptomatic
  —Unrecognized

---

clinical infection. The last category overlaps all the others. **Table 4** summarizes the main clinical manifestations of symptomatic genital herpes.

Primary Herpes Primary herpes is a person's first infection with HSV of either type; by definition, at presentation the patient is seronegative for both HSV-1 and HSV-2. Most cases of primary genital herpes are due to HSV-2, but up to 40% are caused by HSV-1, although this proportion varies widely among various populations. Symptomatic cases of primary genital herpes typically are severe; multiple lesions may persist for 3 weeks or longer, sometimes with recurrent crops of new lesions over the next few weeks. Mucosal involvement is common, with cervicitis in women and urethritis in men. Regional lymphadenopathy usually is present, and systemic manifestations such as headache, fever, and malaise, are frequent. Neuropathic manifestations, such as urinary retention or constipation due to sacral neuropathy, occasionally are seen, and a few patients present with overt meningitis.

Nonprimary Initial Herpes Nonprimary initial herpes results from new infection in a person already infected with the alternate HSV type; acute-phase type-specific serologic testing shows antibody to the previous but not the newly acquired virus type. Almost all cases of nonprimary initial genital herpes are caused by HSV-2 in persons with prior HSV-1 infection. The clinical manifestations generally are less severe than those associated with primary infection but more severe than in recurrent herpes, but the overlap is large. Systemic manifestations, regional lymphadenopathy, and neuropathy are uncommon and, when present, are usually mild. Up to 40% of persons with apparent

Table 4. CLINICAL CHARACTERISTICS OF SYMPTOMATIC GENITAL HERPES

	Clinical Syndrome		
	Primary	Nonprimary	Recurrent
Lesions	Many, bilateral	Fewer	Few, unilateral
Mucosal involvement	Usual	Uncommon	Rare
Lymphadenopathy	Usual	Occasional	Uncommon
Neuropathy*	Common	Uncommon	Rare
Systemic symptoms	Usual	Occasional	Rare
Usual duration	2–4 weeks	1–3 weeks	7–10 days

*Excluding prodromal symptoms

nonprimary initial infection in fact are experiencing the first recognized symptoms of longstanding infection.

Recurrent Herpes Recurrent genital herpes is a person's second or subsequent symptomatic outbreak of herpes due to the same virus type. HSV-2 is responsible for >90% of recurrent genital herpes, because genital HSV-1 is less likely than HSV-2 to cause recurrent outbreaks **(Fig. 3).** Apart from the emotional reactions experienced by many patients, most cases are clinically mild, with only a few lesions. Repeated recurrences usually occur in the same localized area, usually on one side of the body's midline, reflecting the distribution of the dorsal nerve root whose ganglion harbors latent virus. Systemic manifestations, lymphadenopathy, and overt neuropathy usually are absent, although a neuropathic prodrome with paresthesia or dysesthesia sometimes precedes outbreaks.

Subclinical Infection The most important development in the past decade in understanding of the clinical manifestations and epidemiology of genital herpes has been documentation of the frequency of subclinical infection and its contribution to sexual transmission of HSV. Subclinical infection is the most common form of genital herpes, whether primary, nonprimary initial, or recurrent. Subclinical genital herpes occurs both in persons who never had known herpes outbreaks and those who have asymptomatic viral shedding between overt recurrences. Subclinical infection can be truly asymptomatic, but most persons have subtle or atypical symptoms that are not recognized as herpetic. In the NHANES-III survey **(Fig. 2)**, only 9% of persons who were HSV-2-seropositive acknowledged that they had genital herpes. More comprehensive

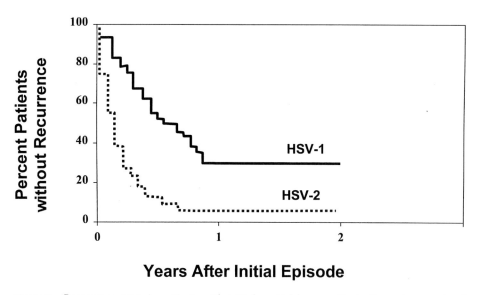

Years After Initial Episode

Figure 3. *Recurrence rates in patients with initial genital herpes, illustrating a lower rate of symptomatic outbreaks in patients infected with HSV-1 than those with HSV-2 infection. Adapted from Corey L, Genital herpes. In: Holmes KK et al,* Sexually Transmitted Diseases, *2d ed. New York, McGraw-Hill, 1990.*

Table 5. PREVALENCE OF HSV-2 DNA IN THE GENITAL TRACT AMONG IMMUNOCOMPETENT MEN AND WOMEN WITH HERPES*

Duration of Sampling (Days)	No. Positive/No. Tested (%)	
	MEN	WOMEN
All Viral Shedding		
30	20/27 (74)	37/42 (88)
40	22/27 (81)	38/42 (90)
50	17/20 (85)	21/22 (95)
Subclinical Shedding Only†		
30	19/27 (70)	35/42 (83)
40	22/27 (81)	36/42 (86)
50	17/20 (85)	20/22 (91)

*Based on daily sampling by polymerase chain reaction, women collected specimens from the vagina, vulva, and anus, and men collected specimens from the urethral meatus, penile skin, and anus. From Wald A, Corey L: unpublished data.
† Limited to days when the subject had no lesions or other symptoms.

questioning typically documents compatible symptoms in 30–40% of patients. However, when HSV-2-seropositive persons are alerted to all possible symptoms of herpes, within several weeks up to two-thirds come to recognize recurrent lesions.

Subclinical viral shedding occurs intermittently in almost all persons infected with HSV-2, at least during the first several years after acquisition. The frequency of subclinical shedding depends on the virus type, the amount of time since the initial infection, the patient's sex, and the type of test used to detect HSV. Just as overt recurrences are less common in genital HSV-1 than HSV-2 infection, subclinical shedding of HSV-1 is much less common than that of HSV-2. Subclinical shedding is somewhat more prevalent in women than men, perhaps because it is easier for men to recognize small penile lesions than for women to perceive painless labial or vaginal ulcers.

Among most women with symptomatic recurrent genital herpes due to HSV-2, during the first year after the initial infection the virus can be detected by culture of the labia, vagina, or anus 5–7% of days when symptoms are absent. When men or women collect specimens from the genitals and anus daily for 2 months, HSV-2 DNA is detected by polymerase chain reaction (PCR) at least once in almost 90% of infected persons **(Table 5).** The frequency of subclinical viral shedding is highest during the first 6 to 12 months after initial infection and declines thereafter, but probably is present at least 1% of days even in persons who have been infected for several years. However, subclinical shedding is neither continuous nor random. During asymptomatic periods, HSV typically can be detected for 2 to 6 consecutive days, followed by longer intervals when tests are continuously negative. **Figure 4** illustrates the viral shedding pattern in typical patients. Many apparently asymptomatic shedding episodes are associated with mild symptoms that patients can learn to recognize. Therefore, patients who are counseled about symptom recognition can detect some (but not all) periods when they are capable of transmitting the infection to sex partners.

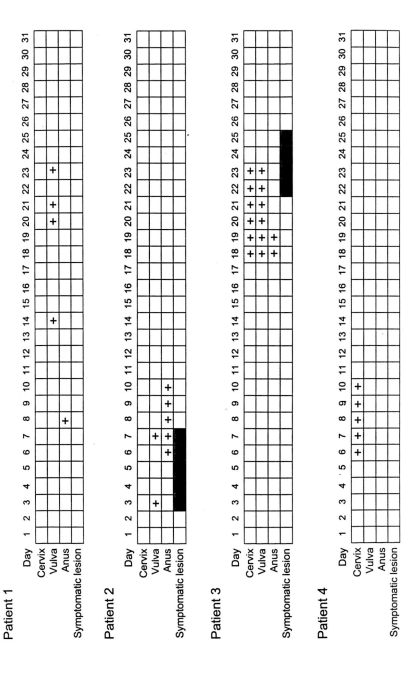

Figure 4. *Shedding of herpes simplex virus type 2 in 4 typical patients with both symptomatic recurrent genital herpes and asymptomatic viral shedding. Adapted from Wald A, et al, N Engl J Med 2000;342:844–50; reprinted with permission.*

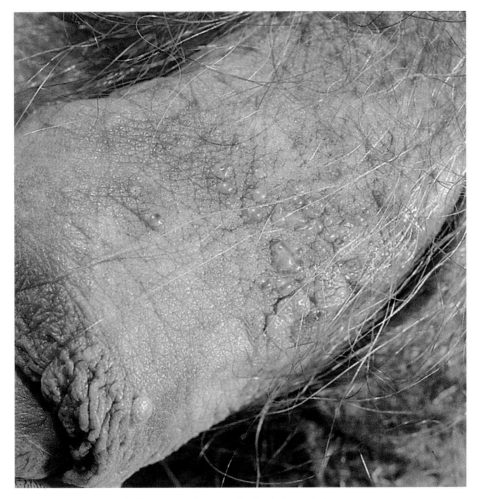

Figure 5. *Primary genital herpes: multiple vesicular lesions of the penis.*

CLINICAL PRESENTATION

Primary Herpes The incubation period typically is 2 to 10 days for symptomatic primary herpes, occasionally up to 3 weeks. Patients usually complain of multiple genital or perianal lesions with increasing pain over 2 to 5 days. **Figures 5–8** illustrate typical lesions in persons with primary genital herpes. Women commonly have prominent

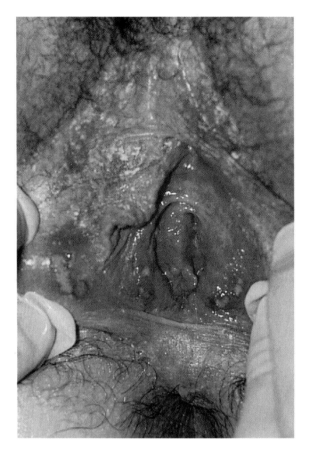

Figure 6. *Primary genital herpes: bilaterally distributed vulvar ulcers. (Courtesy of Claire E. Stevens and Lawrence Corey, MD.)*

"external" dysuria due to urine contacting labial lesions. Herpetic cervicitis **(Fig. 9)** may cause vaginal discharge. Urethritis in men **(Fig. 10)** or women typically causes severe dysuria, and men with herpetic urethritis may complain of urethral discharge. Individual lesions progress over 7 to 14 days from erythematous papules to vesicles containing clear fluid, to pustules, to ulcerated lesions as the epithelium over vesiculopustular lesions erodes, and then to crusted lesions, which is followed by healing. Lesions on mucous membranes or moist cutaneous surfaces (e.g., vulva, urethra, or under the foreskin) often ulcerate early **(Figs. 6 and 8),** usually causing severe pain. Complete healing requires 14 to 21 days, and overlapping crops of new lesions may continue to appear over 3 to 6 weeks.

Many patients with primary herpes complain of inguinal pain or swelling due to regional lymphadenopathy. Urinary retention occasionally occurs, especially in women, due to bladder paralysis resulting from neuropathy involving the sacral nerve roots or to reflex sphincter spasm as a result of severe dysuria. Constipation or anal leakage may occur if sacral neuropathy causes anal sphincter dysfunction. Primary herpetic

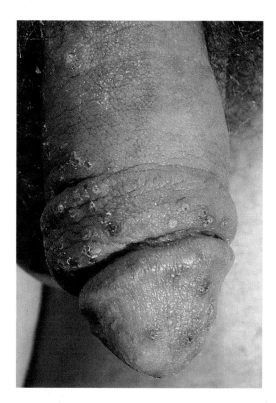

Figure 7. *Primary genital herpes: vesiculopustular and crusted lesions and penile edema.*

proctitis, usually seen in MSM and less frequently in women, causes anorectal pain and often discharge, tenesmus, or rectal bleeding. Fever, myalgias, malaise, and headache are common, and some patients complain of photophobia and stiff neck. The overall severity of symptoms is highly variable. Seroepidemiologic studies indicate that most persons are asymptomatic or have mild or nonspecific symptoms that are not recognized as herpetic.

Nonprimary Initial Herpes Most patients with symptomatic nonprimary initial genital herpes have fewer lesions than those with primary herpes, and the time course is foreshortened. Cervicitis, urethritis, lymphadenopathy, neuropathy, and systemic manifestations are uncommon and, when present, usually are mild. Most patients give a history of sex with a new or possibly infected partner in the preceding 3 weeks. However, up to 40% of persons with apparent nonprimary initial HSV-2 infection have anti-HSV-2 antibody at presentation, indicating that this is the first symptomatic outbreak despite longstanding infection. Some such persons lack histories of sex with a potentially infected partner in the recent past, contributing to the myth that genital herpes sometimes is not sexually acquired.

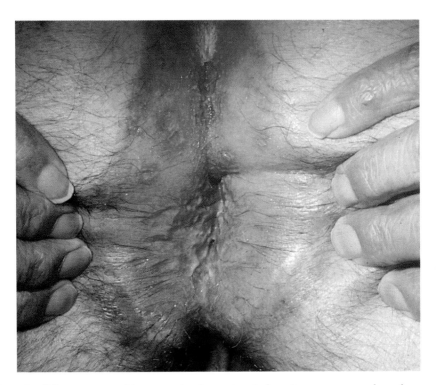

Figure 8. *Primary anorectal herpes: extensive perianal ulcerations; anoscopy showed mucosal ulcers characteristic of herpetic proctitis.*

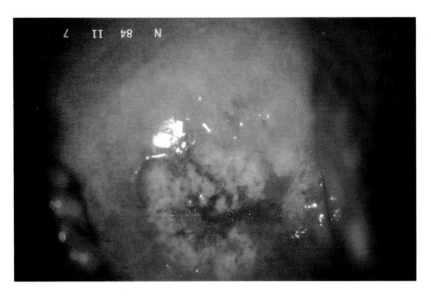

Figure 9. *Primary genital herpes: ulcerative cervicitis. (Courtesy of Claire E. Stevens and Lawrence Corey, MD.)*

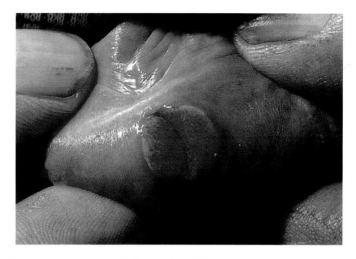

Figure 10. *Primary genital herpes: inflammation of the meatus in a man with herpetic urethritis.*

Recurrent Herpes The hallmark of recurrent genital herpes is a cluster of localized vesiculopustular or ulcerative lesions, lateralized to one side of the midline, that recurs periodically, usually in the same location **(Fig. 11).** However, the presentation is highly variable, and many symptomatic outbreaks lack the classic appearance. Single lesions, small ulcers, or apparent excoriations without a recognized vesiculopustular component, and other "atypical" lesions probably are the most common presentation **(Figs. 12–14).**

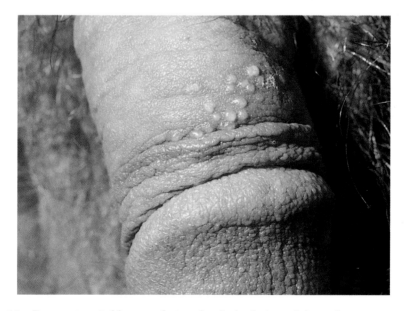

Figure 11. *Recurrent genital herpes: cluster of vesicular lesions of the penis.*

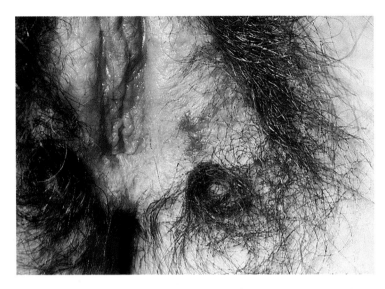

Figure 12. *Recurrent genital herpes: labial ulcer mimicking a traumatic excoriation or other nonspecific lesion.*

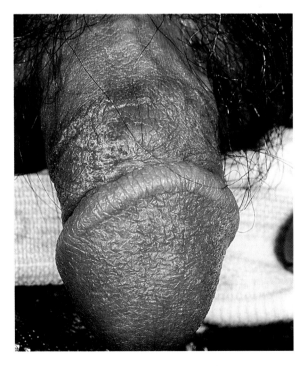

Figure 13. *Recurrent genital herpes: "nonspecific" ulcerative lesion of the penis.*

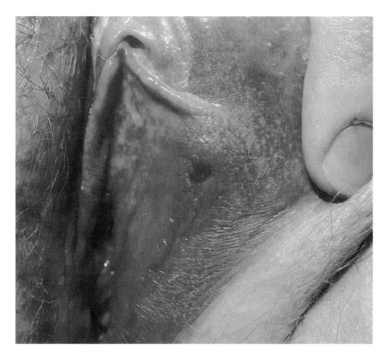

Figure 14. *Recurrent genital herpes: the patient was asymptomatic but subsequently learned to recognize similar recurrent lesions.*

The predominant locations of recurrent herpetic lesions are the glans or shaft of the penis in men and the vaginal introitus, labia minora, or labia majora of women. Anal lesions (and anal subclinical shedding) are common in both sexes, including heterosexual men. Other affected sites include the scrotum, perineum, buttocks, upper thighs, and pubic area; almost any site from the lower abdomen to the thighs may be involved. This distribution reflects the fact that the same sacral nerve may serve the genitals and the anus, buttocks, or other areas. A substantial minority of persons with recurrent herpes experience a neuropathic prodrome of paresthesias or dysesthesias, typically described as a tingling sensation, burning pain, or numbness in the affected area. Prodromal symptoms usually begin 6 to 24 hours before visible lesions appear. Fever, other systemic symptoms, lymphadenopathy, and neuropathic symptoms (aside from the prodrome) are rare; their occurrence suggests initial infection rather than recurrent herpes. In most untreated recurrent outbreaks, pain resolves and lesions begin to heal within 5 days, and the total duration until complete reepithelialization is usually 10 to 12 days.

At least 90% of persons with symptomatic initial HSV-2 infection have symptomatic recurrences, but the frequency is substantially lower among patients with genital HSV-1 infection **(Fig. 3).** Many of the latter experience only one or two outbreaks and none thereafter. After symptomatic initial infection with HSV-2, men have a mean of 5 symptomatic outbreaks and women 4 outbreaks in the next year; almost 40% of patients have 6 or more outbreaks, and about 20% have 10 or more episodes in the first year. Patients with symptomatic recurrences due to HSV-2 generally continue to experience outbreaks for at least a few years, although the average frequency declines slowly. In patients with recurrent genital herpes followed for up to 8 years, the mean decrement in annual recurrence rates was 0.8 outbreak each year. This rate is highly variable and is impossible to predict in any particular patient, but eventually many persons probably cease having recognized outbreaks. Although the time course of subclinical shedding has been less well studied, the frequency clearly declines over time and the course probably is similar to that of symptomatic recurrent herpes.

Complications of Genital Herpes   Erythema multiforme occasionally occurs as an allergic manifestation of recurrent genital or oral herpes, and sometimes can be accompanied by oral mucosal or genital ulceration (Stevens-Johnson syndrome), which may be diagnostically confusing. It is likely that most recurrent erythema multiforme cases in young adults are triggered by genital herpes, which may be subclinical or otherwise undiagnosed. Therefore, diagnostic tests for HSV infection are indicated for all persons with erythema multiforme or Stevens-Johnson syndrome.

Initial oral HSV-1 infection sometimes causes encephalitis or meningoencephalitis, which, if not promptly treated, may be fatal or result in significant neurological deficits. HSV-2 also can infect the central nervous system during primary infection, but in adults it usually causes meningitis without encephalitis. Antiviral therapy speeds recovery of HSV-2 meningitis, and sequelae are rare with or without treatment. HSV-2 causes most cases of the rare syndrome of "benign recurrent lymphocytic meningitis" (Mollaret's meningitis). Such patients have periodic aseptic meningitis, during which HSV-2 DNA can be detected by PCR in the cerebrospinal fluid. In neonatal herpes, either HSV-1 or HSV-2 can cause destructive encephalitis. Type-specific HSV serologic tests, and often virologic tests or PCR to detect HSV, are indicated for all patients with aseptic meningitis or unexplained encephalitis.

HSV infection often is locally aggressive in persons with HIV infection or other forms of cellular immune impairment, but systemic dissemination is rare even in those with advanced immunodeficiency. Prolonged, deeply erosive, painful, debilitating ulcerations commonly involve the anus, genitals, or face **(Figs. 15 and 16),** and HSV-1 sometimes causes ulcerative esophagitis. HSV infection should be routinely sought in HIV-infected patients who have mucocutaneous ulcerations. Despite the aggressive nature of such lesions, antiviral therapy usually is effective both therapeutically and prophylactically.

Neonatal Herpes   Although uncommon, neonatal herpes is the most serious complication of genital herpes, and the potential for its occurrence is one of the main factors that makes herpes frightening to sexually active persons. Two clinical forms are recognized; one is characterized primarily by mucocutaneous herpetic lesions, and the other by various combinations of meningoencephalitis, hepatitis, and consumption coagulopathy, with or without skin or mucous membrane involvement. The initial manifestations in affected newborns often are nonspecific ones such as fever, poor feeding, and failure to thrive. Often these are signs of encephalitis, and even with aggressive antiviral therapy, many infected children suffer devastating sequelae.

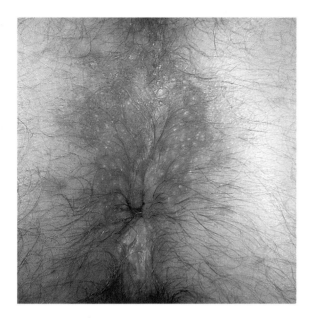

Figure 15. *Erosive perianal lesion due to HSV-2 in a man with AIDS. (Courtesy of Steven J. Medwell, MD.)*

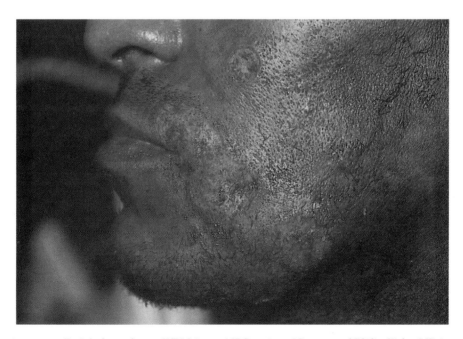

Figure 16. *Facial ulcers due to HSV-1 in an AIDS patient. (Courtesy of Philip Kirby, MD.)*

CLINICAL MANIFESTATIONS OF GENITAL HERPES

PHYSICAL EXAMINATION

Erythematous papules, vesicles, pustules, ulcers, or crusts are seen on examination **(Figs. 5–14)**. Individual lesions usually are 2 to 5 mm in diameter, but all sizes and shapes occur; progression and confluence of lesions sometimes result in irregularly shaped ulcers, especially in primary herpes. Herpetic ulcers generally are not indurated and usually are exquisitely tender. Early ulceration is especially common on moist surfaces and mucous membranes, so that more women than men present with ulcers rather than vesiculopustular or crusted lesions. Many lesions, especially in recurrent herpes, have "nonspecific" appearances, mimicking traumatic lesions, excoriations, folliculitis, and other conditions **(Figs. 12–14)**. The chronic herpetic ulcers associated with AIDS are atypical in comparison to other herpetic lesions, but usually have a consistent appearance with beefy, edematous inflammatory tissue **(Figs. 15 and 16)**.

Herpetic cervicitis is present in most women with primary genital herpes. Unlike mucopurulent cervicitis associated with *Chlamydia trachomatis* or *Neisseria gonorrhoeae*, herpetic cervicitis typically is overtly erosive **(Fig. 9)**. Many men with herpetic urethritis **(Fig. 10)** have localized tenderness of the penis at sites of intraurethral ulcers. If urethral exudate is observed, it typically is scant and mucoid. Acute herpetic proctitis may or may not be associated with vesiculopustular or ulcerative anal lesions **(Fig. 8)**. Digital rectal examination or insertion of an anoscope usually is painful; nevertheless, anoscopy should be attempted because the appearance of mucosal ulcers is diagnostically helpful and direct visualization may improve specimen collection for virologic testing.

Lymphadenopathy, when present, usually is bilateral, firm, and mildly or moderately tender, without fluctuance or overlying cutaneous erythema. Signs of sacral neuropathy include laxity of the anal sphincter and hypesthesia of the genitals, perineum, or other areas served by the sacral nerves. Erythema multiforme is characterized by a typical generalized rash, especially "target" lesions. The oral or genital ulcers of Stevens-Johnson syndrome may be indistinguishable from those caused by HSV itself. The physical findings in meningitis due to HSV (e.g., photophobia, nuchal rigidity) are the same as in cases caused by other viruses, and generally are milder than in bacterial meningitis. Meningitis associated with genital herpes in adults is rarely if ever accompanied by altered consciousness, focal neurologic deficits, seizures, or other signs of encephalitis.

DIFFERENTIAL DIAGNOSIS

The differential diagnosis of genital ulcer disease is broad, but it narrows considerably for sexually active young adults with discrete genital or anal ulcers that are not associated with diffuse genital inflammation (e.g., superficial ulcers associated with yeast vulvovaginitis) and are not merely the genital manifestations of a more widespread dermatosis (e.g., Stevens-Johnson syndrome). In these circumstances, at least 80% of cases are due to genital herpes, syphilis, or chancroid. In virtually all populations and geographic areas of the United States, HSV infection is far more common than syphilis or chancroid; this fact is largely independent of the clinical appearance of the lesions or accompanying lymphadenopathy.

Table 6. ETIOLOGY OF GENITAL ULCER DISEASE AMONG STD CLINIC PATIENTS*

	No. of Patients (%)
Genital herpes†	333 (64.5)
Syphilis†	64 (12.4)
Chancroid	16 (3.1)
PCR negative	116 (22.4)
Total	516

*Based on consecutive patients with genital ulceration attending public STD clinics in 10 U.S. cities, 1996–1997; lesions were tested by polymerase chain reaction (PCR) for DNA of herpes simplex virus, *Treponemal pallidum*, and *Haemophilus ducreyi*. From Mertz K, et al. *J Infect Dis* 1998;178:1795–1798.

†DNA of both *T. pallidum* and HSV was detected in 13 patients, so that 13 (20%) of 64 persons with syphilis also had herpes.

Table 6 summarizes the results of the most recent study of the differential diagnosis of genital ulcer disease in the United States. Patients were selected at STD clinics located in 10 of the 11 cities that then had the highest rates of primary and secondary syphilis, and persons with typical herpes (i.e., vesiculopustular lesions) were excluded. All were tested with a multiplex PCR assay to detect *Treponema pallidum* and *Haemophilus ducreyi*, the causes of syphilis and chancroid, and HSV. Despite the strong selection biases in favor of syphilis and against herpes, genital herpes was the diagnosis in about two-thirds of the patients. Of the 64 patients with syphilis, 13 (20%) also had positive PCR tests for HSV, indicating dual infection.

The presence of a classic chancre of primary syphilis, a nontender, indurated ulcer with a "clean" base **(Figs. 17 and 18),** reliably indicates that disease. However, no other ulcer characteristics are helpful; that is, ulcers of all other appearances are more

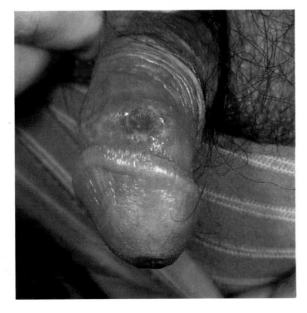

Figure 17. *Primary syphilis: penile chancre.*

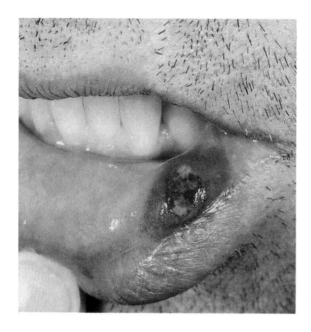

Figure 18. *Primary syphilis: chancre of the lip.*

likely to be herpes than anything else. Chancroid is classically associated with tender ulcers with purulent bases and sometimes undermined edges **(Fig. 19),** but this appearance also is common in herpes **(Figs. 20 and 21).** The nature of the lymphadenopathy often is not helpful, because both syphilis and herpes are associated with mildly tender, firm nodes. Erythema of the overlying skin or fluctuance of the node, however, suggest chancroid, the rare STD lymphogranuloma venereum, or nonsexually transmitted pyogenic infection. Anecdotal experience indicates that even apparently "traumatic" genital ulcers usually are due to herpes. Except when there is an un-

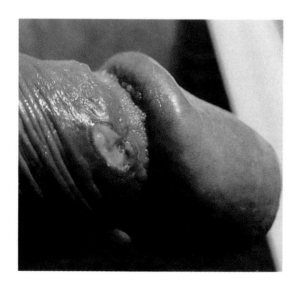

Figure 19. *Chancroid: penile ulcer.*

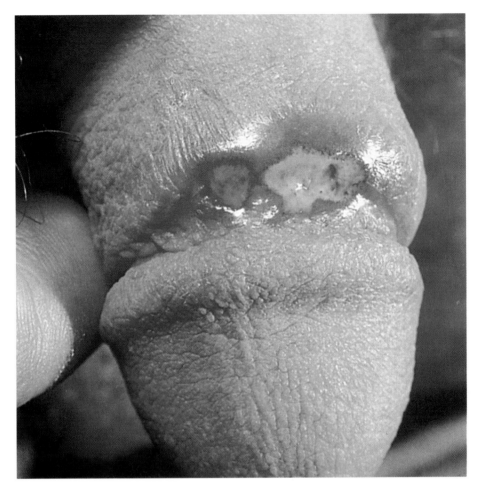

Figure 20. *Primary genital herpes mimicking chancroid.*

equivocal history of trauma at the site of the lesion, such explanations as "I caught it in my zipper" or "I wasn't well lubricated and was injured during sex" often represent assumed explanations by patients who are unaware they have herpes. Thus, failure to perform diagnostic tests for HSV infection results in a missed diagnosis in most young adult patients with genital ulcer disease, regardless of the appearance of the genital lesions. Moreover, substantial minorities of persons with primary syphilis or chancroid are also infected with HSV, as found in the study described above.

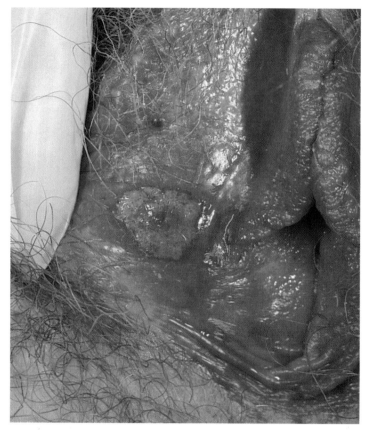

Figure 21. *Vulvar ulcer mimicking chancroid in a woman with initial genital herpes; the small violaceous nodule is an unrelated hemangioma.*

LABORATORY DIAGNOSIS

VIROLOGIC TESTS

As for most infectious diseases, the laboratory diagnosis of HSV infection is based on virologic testing to detect the pathogen itself or on serologic testing to detect specific antibody. In most settings, isolation by cell culture is the virologic test of choice, and culture for HSV is offered by most clinical laboratories in the United States. Culture permits distinction of HSV-1 from HSV-2, which has important implications for prognosis and counseling. The sensitivity of culture is highest for initial episodes of herpes and for testing vesiculopustular or recent ulcerative lesions. The culture yield declines rapidly as lesions begin to heal, as they become nontender, and when lesions of recurrent herpes are more than 2 days old. PCR is substantially more sensitive than culture and is the test of choice when prompt, sensitive diagnosis is critical, such as working up newborns with possible neonatal herpes and whenever cerebrospinal fluid is tested for HSV. Many reference laboratories offer PCR assays, but none is yet commercially available.

Direct fluorescent antibody (FA) tests for HSV are almost as sensitive as culture, but do not differentiate the two HSV types. Microscopy of Papanicolaou smears or Giemsa-stained scrapings of lesions to detect multinucleated giant cells typical of herpes (the Tzanck test) is both insensitive and nonspecific; it is indicated rarely, if ever. A report of possible HSV infection on a routine Pap smear is nonspecific and, therefore, unreliable; no patient should be definitively diagnosed as having genital herpes on the basis of a routine cervical cytology test, although such a result should lead to performance of a more specific diagnostic test.

SEROLOGY

Type-specific serology is a mainstay of diagnosis of HSV infection and has important roles in counseling to prevent both sexual and perinatal transmission. The HSV antibody tests historically offered by most laboratories, typically based on indirect immunofluorescence, complement fixation, or neutralization technologies, do not distinguish antibody to HSV-1 from that to HSV-2, despite manufacturers' or laboratories' assertions that they do so. Some such tests are especially misleading because the results are presented as titers of HSV-1 and HSV-2 antibody that seem to indicate definitive, quantitative results. A positive result with such a test reliably indicates infection with HSV, and a negative result reliably excludes HSV infection if performed >3 months after acquisition. However, because more than one-half of all adults are HSV-1 seropositive, a positive test is useless in evaluating patients with possible genital herpes. In addition, determining whether such antibodies include immunoglobulin G (IgG) or immunoglobulin M (IgM) provides little or no useful information. IgM antibody often is present in recurrent genital herpes, and its presence does not necessarily denote recently acquired infection.

For 15 years, HSV glycoprotein G-based assays that accurately differentiate HSV-1 from HSV-2 antibody using Western blot or other technologies were available in a few research or reference laboratories, but their expense and technical considerations limited their availability. More recently, type-specific antibody tests based on HSV glycoprotein G finally came to market. Their availability has greatly improved the prospects for accurate diagnosis of genital herpes. Compared with Western blot, the gold standard of serologic assay, the new tests have specificities of >98% for detection of HSV-2 antibody and sensitivities of 90–95%, depending on the population studied and assay conditions. One rapid, office-based HSV-2 antibody test gives results in a few minutes. To avoid confusing results from tests that are called type-specific but are not, clinicians ordering HSV serologic tests should specify that a glycoprotein G-based test be done, or should request a particular test by name. (Note that *glycoprotein G* is distinct from *immunoglobulin G*, or IgG.) **Table 7** lists the commercially available assays that were approved by the U.S. Food and Drug Administration at the time of writing.

The positive predictive value of a diagnostic test—i.e., the likelihood that a positive result is accurate—depends not only on test performance, but also on the probability (before testing) of infection in the patient. Therefore, effective use of the type-specific HSV antibody tests depends on the clinical setting. They are diagnostically useful in persons with a high likelihood of HSV-2 infection, such as those with symptoms sug-

Table 7. GLYCOPROTEIN G-BASED TYPE-SPECIFIC SEROLOGICAL TESTS FOR ANTIBODY TO HERPES SIMPLEX VIRUS TYPES 1 AND 2*

Test	Manufacturer	Comment†
Western blot	Reference laboratories	The definitive test; sensitivity ≥95%, specificity 100%; available at selected research or reference laboratories
HerpeSelect HSV-1 and HSV-2 ELISA‡	Focus Technologies§	Sensitivity ~90%
HerpeSelect HSV-1 and HSV-2 immunoblot	Focus Technologies§	Uses same antigens as Focus ELISA tests; sensitivity ~90%
POCKit	Diagnology, Inc	Point-of-care test, giving result in <10 minutes; detects HSV-2 antibody only; sensitivity 90–95%

*Commercially available at time of writing; other assays are in development and likely to come to market in coming years. Use of trade and manufacturers' names is for identification only and does not imply endorsement by the author.

†Sensitivity and specificity figures are for detection of HSV-2 antibody in patients tested ≥3 months after acquisition of HSV-2 infection.

‡ELISA denotes enzyme-linked immunoabsorbant assay.

§Formerly Microbiology Reference Laboratory (MRL).

gestive of genital herpes and for the sex partners of infected persons, and they should be liberally used in evaluating such patients. The tests' utility for other purposes, such as screening asymptomatic populations with lower prevalences of infection, may depend on the availability of supplemental testing to confirm positive results. The historically validated confirmatory serological test is the HSV Western blot, available in a few reference laboratories, such as the University of Washington Clinical Laboratories, Seattle, Washington.

DIAGNOSTIC APPROACH

Table 8 summarizes a practical approach to diagnosis of genital ulcer disease in sexually active young adults or others at high risk of genital herpes. A diagnosis based only on the history and physical examination often is reliable in classic genital herpes, especially for primary herpes and in patients who present with typical lesions such as vesicles, pustules, or a cluster of superficial ulcers. Nevertheless, laboratory confirmation of the diagnosis is recommended even in these cases to determine virus type and to provide an unequivocal diagnosis because of the psychological stress associated with herpes. Screening tests for other STDs, such as chlamydial infection, gonorrhea, syphilis, and HIV, also are indicated for all patients with newly acquired herpes.

Table 8. DIAGNOSTIC TESTS IN GENITAL ULCER DISEASE

- Typical genital herpes (vesiculopustular lesions)
  - —Culture for HSV* (optional†)
  - —Type-specific HSV serology (if culture negative)
- Uncertain clinical diagnosis or atypical presentation
  - —Culture for HSV*
  - —Type-specific HSV serology
  - —Serologic test for syphilis
- Selected patients‡
  - —Convalescent type-specific HSV serology (6–12 weeks)
  - —Darkfield examination for *Treponemal pallidum*
  - —Culture for *Haemophilus ducreyi*
  - —Culture for pyogenic bacteria
  - —Biopsy

*Direct fluorescent antibody (FA) test may be substituted if culture is not available, but does not distinguish between HSV-1 and HSV-2; polymerase chain reaction (PCR) test is more sensitive, but not commercially available in most settings.

†HSV virologic testing may be considered optional for purely diagnostic purposes if the clinical manifestations are typical, but patient anxiety and the need to determine the HSV type usually warrants definitive laboratory diagnosis.

‡If preceding evaluation nondiagnostic or if clinical or epidemiologic features suggest syphilis, chancroid, or other diagnosis.

A virologic test for HSV is definitely indicated in all patients with genital ulcers other than classic genital herpes. Culture (or PCR, if available) is recommended; a direct FA test may be used if culture is not available. No virologic test is, however, 100% sensitive, especially for dry or healing lesions, and a negative result usually does not exclude HSV infection with certainty. Therefore, many experts recommend that both culture and a type-specific serological test for HSV-2 be done routinely in all patients with genital ulcer disease or other clinical suspicion of genital herpes. A serologic test for syphilis should be done in all patients with genital ulceration that is not typical for herpes, because syphilis is the second most frequent cause of genital ulcer disease in sexually active young persons. Either the Venereal Disease Research Laboratory (VDRL) test or rapid plasma reagin (RPR) test is appropriate.

If initial genital herpes is suspected and both culture and the serologic test are negative, a convalescent type-specific serologic test (at least 6 weeks and preferably 3 months after presentation) may establish the diagnosis. In addition, the clinician should see the patient within 24 hours for repeat culture in the event symptoms recur. Patients with genital ulcers whose morphology suggests syphilis or chancroid, and other patients in whom the workup for HSV infection is negative, should be referred for darkfield microscopy or direct FA test for *T. pallidum* and culture for *H. ducreyi*. Testing for *T. pallidum* is available at most public health laboratories and clinics, and some public health or reference laboratories can isolate *H. ducreyi*. If the diagnosis remains obscure, biopsy and other special tests may be required to exclude rare conditions, such as Behçet's syndrome **(Fig. 22),** cancer, and other diseases.

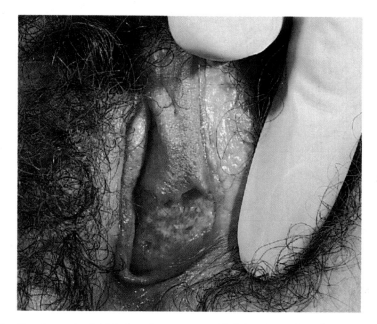

Figure 22. *Deeply erosive labial ulcer in a woman with Behçet's syndrome.*

TREATMENT

The mainstays of management of patients with genital herpes are antiviral therapy and personal counseling, and both are indicated in most patients. Counseling has two broad goals: (1) to ameliorate the psychological impact of infection, and (2) to reduce the risk of sexual and perinatal transmission of HSV.

PRINCIPLES OF ANTIHERPETIC CHEMOTHERAPY

The main antiherpetic drugs are acyclovir and its pro-drug valacyclovir, and penciclovir and its pro-drug famciclovir. Acyclovir was the first effective, nontoxic, systemic antiviral drug; its developer earned the Nobel Prize. Acyclovir and penciclovir themselves lack antiviral activity; the enzyme thymidine kinase, produced only by herpes virus-infected cells and required by HSV for replication, mediates the first stage of phosphorylation of the compound, which is then completed by cellular enzymes **(Fig. 23)**. Acyclovir triphosphate or penciclovir triphosphate halts HSV DNA replication. Because the parent drugs are not phosphorylated in the absence of HSV-induced thymidine kinase, they do not interfere with DNA replication in normal mammalian cells, partly explaining their lack of toxicity.

Acyclovir has poor bioavailability; only about 20% of the drug is absorbed after oral administration. Valacyclovir, the valine ester of acyclovir, is well absorbed after oral administration, after which de-esterification releases free acyclovir. Thus, oral valacyclovir delivers higher blood levels of acyclovir with reduced dosing frequency. Like acyclovir, penciclovir is poorly absorbed after oral administration; famciclovir is a pro-

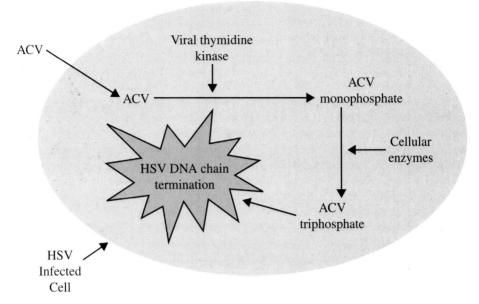

Figure 23. *Schematic representation of the mechanism of action of acyclovir. ACV denotes acyclovir. The metabolism and action of penciclovir are as shown for acyclovir.*

drug ester that enhances its bioavailability. Acyclovir itself is available in parenteral and topical formulations, as well as orally, and penciclovir is available as a topical preparation.

Acyclovir in sufficiently large doses usually is effective, but nonetheless low blood levels occasionally result in suboptimal clinical responses. Aside from the improved bioavailability of valacyclovir and famciclovir, there are no other overriding advantages or disadvantages of any of these drugs over the others, and the therapeutic choice can be based on ancillary factors, such as dosing convenience and cost. The FDA-approved oral acyclovir regimens require dosing 5 times daily, but the drug's pharmacokinetics and clinical experience support twice daily or three times daily administration. Valacyclovir has the advantage of once daily dosing for suppressive therapy. Acyclovir, valacyclovir, and famciclovir cause few side effects or toxicity; the frequencies of headache, mildly abnormal liver function tests, and other nonspecific effects are similar in patients taking active drug or placebo. Allergic reactions are very rare to all three drugs.

Resistance of HSV to acyclovir and penciclovir is rare, and to date has been almost entirely limited to persons with AIDS who were taking suppressive antiherpetic therapy. The most common type of resistance develops when HSV ceases to produce thymidine kinase. However, thymidine kinase–negative HSV mutants may have reduced virulence, and there is only one reported case of de novo acquisition of resistant HSV. Moreover, after cessation of treatment for a few weeks, fully sensitive thymidine kinase–producing HSV often reemerges in the infected person and therapeutic efficacy returns. For patients with clinically significant infection with acyclovir-resistant HSV, systemic foscarnet or topical cidofovir often are effective. Mathematical modeling suggests that the likelihood of widespread, clinically significant resistance of HSV to acyclovir and penciclovir is low, even with high rates of treatment in the general population.

Topical therapy of genital herpes has little or no role in management. Topical acyclovir or penciclovir slightly speeds the time until lesion cultures for HSV become negative, but clinical resolution is no more rapid than in patients given placebo. All persons with genital herpes of sufficient clinical severity or psychological impact to warrant treatment should be offered systemic therapy. Many "natural" remedies such as lysine, arginine, vitamins, herbal extracts, and dietary manipulations have been promoted for the treatment of genital herpes, but few have theoretical rationales to suggest possible efficacy and none has been shown to be effective in controlled trials, whether for prevention, therapy, or suppression of recurrences. None is recommended for routine management.

TREATMENT REGIMENS

Clinicians should have a low threshold for recommending and prescribing antiviral therapy for patients with genital herpes. The drugs are benign, and many patients, including some who initially seem not to be disturbed by the diagnosis, will experience benefits in well-being and reduced stress and depression, sometimes out of proportion to the objective clinical benefit. The author's treatment recommendations are summarized in **Table 9.**

Initial Genital Herpes Antiviral therapy is indicated for most patients with initial genital herpes, whether primary or nonprimary. Even those who present with mild manifestations are at substantial risk for prolonged symptoms and for increasing severity over the next 1 to 2 weeks. Valacyclovir, famciclovir, or acyclovir are given for 10 days in the doses shown in **Table 9.** In the past, it was recommended that patients with acute

---

Table 9. RECOMMENDED ANTIVIRAL DRUG REGIMENS FOR TREATMENT OF GENITAL HERPES*

- Initial infection
  - —Valacyclovir 1.0 g PO *bid* for 10 days
  - —Famciclovir 250 mg PO *tid* for 10 days
  - —Acyclovir 400 mg PO *tid* (or 200 mg PO 5 times daily) for 10 days

- Recurrent infection, episodic therapy
  - —Valacyclovir 500 mg PO *bid* for 3 days†
  - —Famciclovir 125 mg PO *bid* for 5 days
  - —Acyclovir 400 mg PO *tid* (or 200 mg PO 5 times daily) for 5 days

- Recurrent infection, suppressive therapy
  - —Valacyclovir 500 mg PO daily‡
  - —Famciclovir 250 mg PO *bid*
  - —Acyclovir 400 mg PO *bid*

---

*Author's recommendations, adapted from 2001 STD treatment guidelines, Centers for Disease Control and Prevention (in press).

†Only valacyclovir has been documented to be effective when given for 3 days, but 3-day regimens of famciclovir and acyclovir are also likely to be effective.

‡The dose of valacyclovir should be increased to 1.0 g daily in patients with ≥10 symptomatic recurrences per year.

herpetic proctitis or initial oral herpes receive higher doses of acyclovir (e.g., 800 mg PO *tid*), but no data support the need for higher doses and most experts prescribe the standard regimens. Intravenous acyclovir (5–10 mg/kg body weight every 8 hours) is used for rare patients with illness sufficiently severe to require hospitalization; once clinical improvement is observed, usually after 2 to 5 days, treatment can be switched to an oral regimen to complete 10 days total therapy.

In most patients with initial herpes, onset of new lesions ceases within 2 days of starting treatment; soon thereafter fever and systemic manifestations begin to resolve, and healing usually is well underway within 4 to 5 days. A few patients given oral acyclovir may have suboptimal clinical responses because of the drug's poor bioavailability; they may be managed by switching to valacyclovir or famciclovir, or by doubling the dose of acyclovir.

Recurrent Genital Herpes   Recurrent herpes can be treated either with episodic treatment of individual outbreaks or with suppressive therapy to prevent recurrences. Episodic therapy is effective only if begun within 24 hours of onset of an outbreak. Therefore, patients on episodic therapy should retain a supply of drug to facilitate immediate therapy when symptoms begin. Even with prompt onset, the efficacy of episodic therapy is modest in most patients; the time to cessation of pain and onset of healing typically is accelerated by only 1 to 2 days. However, treatment is more effective in some patients, and sometimes prompt treatment at onset of prodrome or before vesicles develop can abort the development of mature lesions. Episodic therapy probably is most useful for patients with relatively infrequent recurrences, perhaps especially those whose outbreaks are atypically severe or prolonged.

Suppressive antiviral therapy can be administered to prevent symptomatic outbreaks. Treatment should be initiated with one of the regimens shown in **Table 9,** but the dose or frequency may then be adjusted to balance efficacy, convenience, and cost. The frequency of symptomatic outbreaks is reduced by 70–80%, but if breakthrough episodes occur, they often are brief, so the reduction in symptomatic days may be greater. About one-half of the patients on suppressive therapy report complete abolition of symptomatic recurrences. Suppressive therapy has been studied primarily in patients who have 6 or more recurrences per year, but many persons with fewer recurrences, especially those with significant stress or depression, also benefit.

Recent studies demonstrate marked improvement in quality of life and reduced psychological consequences of genital herpes as a result of suppressive therapy. Therefore, suppressive therapy should be discussed with all patients with recurrent herpes and offered to most of them. In addition, persons with initial genital herpes should be informed about the availability and efficacy of suppressive therapy, in case they have recurrent outbreaks. Knowing that suppressive therapy is available for future outbreaks sometimes helps patients cope with the initial diagnosis. Because genital herpes recurs most frequently in the first several months after initial infection, and suppression of chronic recurrent herpes improves quality of life, a controlled trial is underway to assess the psychological and quality-of-life benefits of initiating suppressive therapy immediately after treatment of initial genital herpes.

Suppressive treatment should be interrupted periodically (e.g., once a year) to reassess the frequency of recurrences, the psychological impact of the disease, and the need to continue therapy. There is no increased severity or frequency of recurrences after cessation of treatment ("rebound effect"), even after several years of suppressive therapy, despite a common belief to the contrary.

In addition to preventing symptomatic recurrences of genital herpes, suppressive treatment reduces the frequency of subclinical viral shedding, suggesting a possible role in preventing sexual transmission. However, subclinical shedding is not entirely eliminated, and some potential for transmission probably persists on therapy. The results of a nationwide, multicenter trial of valacyclovir to prevent transmission in herpes-discordant couples are likely to be available by 2003. Until these results are known, patients should be informed that the efficacy of valacyclovir and other antiherpetic drugs in preventing transmission is unknown, and treatment should not be prescribed specifically to prevent transmission.

Treatment of Pregnant Women   Acyclovir, valacyclovir, and famciclovir probably are safe for pregnant women and fetuses, although none is approved by the U.S. Food and Drug Administration for use during pregnancy. For over a decade, the manufacturer of acyclovir maintained a registry of women who inadvertently received the drug while pregnant. The incidence of congenital anomalies and other adverse outcomes was low, consistent with historical controls, and no adverse pregnancy outcomes have been attributed to the drug. However, too few persons were treated and followed to exclude the possibility of rare adverse effects. Few data are available on the safety of valacyclovir or famciclovir during pregnancy.

Most experts agree that pregnant women with initial genital herpes should be treated with acyclovir, but experience with valacyclovir and famciclovir is limited. Standard doses of acyclovir **(Table 9)** may be used, except that intravenous administration may be preferred during labor for women who have initial genital herpes at term. Giving suppressive acyclovir therapy during the last month of pregnancy to women with symptomatic recurrent herpes may prevent otherwise unnecessary cesarean sections by reducing the likelihood of an outbreak of herpes near term. Such treatment is now recommended by some experts for women with symptomatic recurrent herpes, and its use is endorsed (but not specifically advised) by the American College of Obstetrics and Gynecology.

Neonatal Herpes   The overriding principle in the treatment of neonatal herpes is to maintain a low threshold for antiviral therapy and to start treatment early. The recommended regimen is acyclovir 20 mg/kg body weight IV every 8 hours for 14 to 21 days. Patients should be managed in consultation with a pediatric infectious diseases specialist or other expert. Because acyclovir is nontoxic and even a brief delay in treatment may result in neurologic sequelae or death, acyclovir should be administered promptly whenever the disease is expected. Some experts recommend that IV acyclovir be given prophylactically to babies born to mothers with initial genital herpes during delivery, but such treatment probably is not indicated for infants born to women with recurrent herpes, even if lesions are present during delivery.

SUPPORTIVE THERAPY

Patients with genital herpes should be advised to keep lesions clean and dry by washing the affected area 2 to 3 times daily, wearing loose-fitting cotton underwear, and perhaps sprinkling cornstarch in underwear; these measures may be especially helpful in women. Topical anesthetic ointments may help control pain. Sometimes nonsteroidal anti-inflammatory drugs or opiates may be helpful in limiting pain, and, in the author's experience, phenazopyridine helps some patients with dysuria.

COUNSELING

Anticipating, recognizing, and ameliorating the personal impact and psychological consequences of genital herpes and taking steps to prevent sexual and perinatal transmission are integral to management. Patients with newly acquired herpes have many concerns, which vary greatly between patients and over time in individuals; some of the chief ones are listed in **Table 10.**

The first step in counseling is to provide accurate information about all aspects of the disease. Because the emotional impact of the diagnosis and often the severity of symptoms will prevent many patients from absorbing comprehensive advice, counseling at the time of diagnosis often can be quite brief. The provider should assure that the patient understands that:

- Effective symptomatic treatment is available.
- If the patient experiences symptomatic recurrences, they probably will be milder than the initial episode.
- In the event of recurrences, effective preventive therapy is available.
- Although the infection was acquired sexually, the patient's partner likely did not know that he or she has herpes, or believed that he or she was not infectious when exposure occurred.

The provider should ascertain the patient's other chief concerns or fears and briefly address them, but extended counseling usually should be deferred to a follow-up visit. Most patients will not perceive or articulate all their concerns at the initial visit, and many will forget some of the clinician's responses. In any case, few clinicians have the time to provide all the answers in the detail desired by some patients, especially if

Table 10. COMMON CONCERNS OF PATIENTS WITH NEWLY DIAGNOSED GENITAL HERPES

- Pain and other clinical manifestations
- Fear of recurrent outbreaks
- Fear of transmitting infection to sex partners
- Fear of nonsexual transmission to other persons
- Impact on current sexual relationship or on forming new ones
- Belief that a sex partner has been unfaithful
- Belief that a partner knowingly failed to disclose his or her herpes infection
- Fear of neonatal infection
- Belief that herpes in women requires all subsequent pregnancies to be delivered by cesarean section
- Fear of cervical cancer
- Fear of the elevated risk of HIV transmission or acquisition
- Shame, guilt, and/or sense of contamination, contagion, or uncleanness

the diagnosis was not anticipated and time was not allotted for counseling at the initial visit. Accordingly, sufficient time should be scheduled at a follow-up visit to address the patient's concerns. Patients may be given brochures or other written information about genital herpes, as well as additional sources of accurate information about the disease such as Internet web sites and telephone hotlines. These can significantly shorten the follow-up visit and provide structure to subsequent counseling. Many such resources are available, and selected ones are summarized in the Appendix. The elements of counseling to prevent HSV transmission are described below.

PREVENTION

Clinicians have important roles in ensuring that their patients with genital herpes and other patients at risk for the disease understand ways to prevent transmission to other persons, and in promulgating a public health perspective toward this most public of infectious diseases.

PERSONAL STRATEGIES TO PREVENT GENITAL HERPES

Sexually active young persons have two main strategies at their disposal to prevent transmitting or acquiring genital herpes (and all STDs): (1) abstention from sex when herpetic lesions are present, and (2) use of condoms. Abstaining when lesions are present requires awareness of the diagnosis and its symptoms, including subtle ones. Even though transmission also occurs as a result of subclinical viral shedding, the likelihood of infecting a sex partner clearly is reduced to the extent that infected persons avoid sex during some infectious periods. In many HSV-2-discordant couples, transmission to the susceptible partner is delayed many years, sometimes indefinitely, by avoiding sex during symptomatic outbreaks.

Consistent use of condoms reduces the risk of transmission in HSV-2-discordant couples but does not eliminate it. Recent data suggest that condoms reduce transmission from men to women more effectively than from women to men, but properly used condoms probably reduce transmission in either direction. The partial effectiveness of condoms almost certainly reflects the occasional occurrence of herpetic lesions (or sites of subclinical viral shedding) that are not covered by condoms, or the spread of con-taminated secretions to the rim of the condom due to sliding of the penis within the condom. There is no evidence that HSV can pass through an intact condom. Condoms are variably accepted, and of course consistent use is incompatible with conception in those couples seeking to start a family. Nevertheless, condoms should be advocated as useful protection against transmission, especially during the first 6 to 12 months after initial genital herpes, when both clinical recurrences and subclinical shedding are most frequent. It seems likely that the female condom, by providing wider anatomic coverage, may be more effective than the male condom, but no data are available, and the female condom has not gained wide acceptance.

Another theoretically effective strategy to prevent genital herpes is to select sex partners with like HSV serological status. This approach clearly is impractical on a wide scale, but personal advertisements in printed media and on the Internet illustrate that some persons pursue this strategy, and type-specific serological tests occasionally may be requested by patients for this purpose. A final theoretical strategy, unacceptable to almost all persons, is permanent sexual abstinence.

MANAGEMENT AND COUNSELING OF SEX PARTNERS

In most settings, the practicing clinician encounters two categories of couples with genital herpes. In the first, the patient presents with initial genital herpes, acquired from a known partner. The second common situation involves a monogamous couple in which one partner has longstanding genital herpes and the other apparently does not, and the couple wishes to prevent transmission in the fetus.

New Acquisition of Genital Herpes   This situation may involve either an ongoing sexual partnership or a new one. In either case, the source of the patient's infection is clear. Typically, the source partner either was unaware that he or she had HSV infection or knew herpes was present but believed he or she was not infectious when exposure occurred. Sometimes, of course, a source contact has ignored a known potential for transmission, but such cases are in the minority.

Table 11 summarizes an approach to counseling the couple in which one person has newly acquired herpes. The virus type in the newly infected partner, if not yet known, should be established by culture or a type-specific serological test. The source partner should be examined, counseled about the likelihood of infection or, if genital or oral herpes is known to be present, about subclinical viral shedding and the potential for transmission between symptomatic episodes. If the source partner is not known to have HSV infection, he or she should have a type-specific serological test and should be counseled to recognize symptoms of herpes, however subtle, and a viral culture should be obtained when lesions appear.

In most such cases, the partner named as the source of the patient's infection will have HSV infection of the same type as the patient. If the relationship is likely to continue, both persons should be given the reassuring information that they are mutually infected with the same HSV type, further transmission will not occur, and steps to prevent transmission are unimportant, except as necessary to avoid pain or discomfort during sex. However, if the source patient is likely to have other sex partners, he or she should be counseled about strategies to prevent transmission.

When genital herpes first appears in one partner of a mutually monogamous couple, they should be told that infection does not necessarily imply that either partner has

---

Table 11.   COUNSELING AND MANAGEMENT OF COUPLES IN WHICH ONE PERSON ACQUIRES INITIAL GENITAL HERPES

- Determine HSV type in the newly infected person, using viral culture and/or type-specific serological testing
- Examine and counsel partner
- Type-specific serological test of sex partner
- Counsel partner about strategies to prevent transmission to future sex partners

---

been unfaithful. It also does not imply nonsexual acquisition of the virus, because the newly symptomatic partner might be experiencing the first recognized outbreak months or years after the initial infection; alternatively, transmission sometimes first occurs after many months or years of mutual monogamy.

Herpes-Discordant Couples The more common situation in most clinical practices involves a couple in an ongoing relationship in which one person has longstanding genital herpes and wishes to avoid transmission to the other partner **(Table 12).** The first step is to determine the HSV type in the infected person by viral culture or a type-specific serological test. The clinician should take a careful history of the apparently uninfected person to elicit symptoms compatible with genital or oral herpes. A type-specific serological test should be done. If serological testing confirms that the asymptomatic partner is infected with the same HSV type, the couple can be reassured; no precautions against transmission are required, and in the event of pregnancy, cesarean section is unlikely to be necessary.

If serological testing confirms that the asymptomatic partner is not infected with the same virus type as the index patient, the couple should be counseled about the substantial efficacy of using condoms and avoiding sex when the infected person is symptomatic and about the risk of transmission from subclinical shedding. In addition to learning ways to avoid transmission, herpes-discordant couples should be told that if transmission occurs, the newly infected person may experience few or no symptoms (because subclinical infection is common), and that effective antiviral therapy is available if symptomatic initial infection occurs. This information can help reduce a cou-

Table 12. COUNSELING AND MANAGEMENT OF HERPES-DISCORDANT MONOGAMOUS COUPLES

- Determine HSV type in the infected partner using viral culture or type-specific serology
- Evaluate the apparently uninfected partner
  —History of past genital herpes diagnosis and symptoms
  —Type-specific HSV serological test
- If serology shows partner infected with same HSV type as index patient
  —No precautions necessary to prevent transmission
  —Consider avoiding sex when symptomatic partner has outbreaks, as needed for comfort
  —Low risk for neonatal transmission; in event of pregnancy, cesarean section probably will not be required
- If serological test shows partner *not* infected with same HSV type as index patient
  —Partner is susceptible
  —Transmission risk will be reduced by avoiding sex when index patient has symptoms
  —Infection can occur through subclinical shedding
  —Consistent use of condoms will reduce (but not eliminate) risk of transmission
  —Herpes does not preclude healthy, rewarding sex
  —If transmission occurs despite these precautions, symptoms may be mild or absent, and effective treatment is available
  —Importance of avoiding transmission to the woman if she becomes pregnant

ple's anxiety about transmission. The couple should understand that genital herpes rarely is a serious impediment to healthy, pleasurable, and mutually rewarding sex. Finally, if the man in a heterosexual herpes-discordant couple is infected, the couple must be counseled to avoid sex (genital sex if the index case is infected with HSV-2, orogenital contact if HSV-1) during the third trimester of current or future pregnancies.

PUBLIC HEALTH STRATEGIES FOR HERPES PREVENTION

For most STDs, clinicians understand and invoke standard principles of public health when they manage their patients. Screening tests are done in asymptomatic persons at risk for chlamydial infection, gonorrhea, syphilis, or HIV infection; patients are advised that their partners should be evaluated and treated; and cases are reported to health authorities if required by local statute. However, the public health aspects of genital herpes have largely been ignored, perhaps even more by public health agencies than by some clinicians. This situation is starting to change. Although the structure and role of a national genital herpes prevention effort is uncertain, the clinician should employ many of the same strategies they take for granted for other STDs.

A public health approach to genital herpes is summarized in **Table 13,** and many of the elements are implied in the discussion on counseling. Virologic tests for HSV should be performed in all sexually active patients with genital ulceration; without testing for HSV, most cases of herpes will be missed and the etiology of genital ulceration will remain obscure. Glycoprotein G-based type-specific serological tests for HSV should be used liberally to help in the diagnosis of genital ulcer disease, to evaluate the asymptomatic sex partners of persons with genital herpes, and to assess patients who are concerned they may have herpes and request an evaluation for it.

Type-specific serological testing of pregnant women and, if seronegative, their husbands or other sex partners can help prevent neonatal herpes. Although routine, widespread application of this strategy should await further studies of its practical utility

---

Table 13. PUBLIC HEALTH APPROACH TO MANAGEMENT AND PREVENTION OF GENITAL HERPES

- Routine virologic testing for HSV diagnosis in patients with genital ulceration
- Liberal use of type-specific HSV serological tests
  - —Sex partners of persons with genital herpes
  - —Patients with symptoms consistent with genital herpes
  - —Patient request to evaluate for genital herpes
  - —Selected pregnant women and their sex partners
- Consider antiviral therapy of selected pregnant women with recurrent genital herpes to prevent cesarean delivery
- Counsel infected persons and their sex partners
  - —Symptom recognition
  - —Subclinical viral shedding
  - —Condoms

---

and cost-effectiveness, such testing clearly is indicated in pregnant women whose current or past sex partners are believed to have genital herpes, so that discordant couples (uninfected woman, infected partner) can be counseled to avoid exposure during the third trimester. Specifically, HSV-2-seronegative women should be counseled to avoid intercourse in the last trimester with men known or suspected to have HSV-2 infection or genital herpes; and HSV-1-seronegative women should avoid cunnilingus, especially with a partner believed to have oral herpes or HSV-1 infection. Clinicians should consider the use of antiviral therapy during the last month of pregnancy for pregnant women with symptomatic recurrent genital herpes to prevent otherwise unnecessary cesarean sections. Surveillance cultures for HSV in pregnant women are not effective in preventing neonatal herpes and are not recommended. Finally, the clinician should routinely counsel infected persons, their sex partners, and other sexually active persons about symptom recognition, subclinical viral shedding, and the personal prevention strategies to avoid HSV transmission.

Immunization has long been a hope for prevention of genital herpes and other HSV infections, but to date no vaccines have been unequivocally effective. A recently completed multicenter study showed a candidate vaccine to modestly reduce the risk of HSV-2 infection in HSV-1-negative women, but not in men or HSV-1-seronegative women. Although new vaccine candidates are in development and immunization may hold promise in the future, effective vaccines against HSV are not likely to be commercially available for at least several years.

ANNOTATED REFERENCES

GENERAL REVIEWS

Centers for Disease Control and Prevention. 1998 Guidelines for treatment of sexually transmitted diseases. *Morbid Mortal Weekly Rep* 1998;47(RR-1). *CDC's treatment guidelines, including recommendations for prevention strategies; updated guidelines will be published in 2001.*

Corey L, Wald A. Genital herpes. In: Holmes KK, et al, *Sexually Transmitted Diseases*, 3d ed. New York, McGraw-Hill, 1999:285–312. *An excellent overview of genital herpes in the premier STD textbook.*

Handsfield HH. Genital herpes. In: Handsfield HH, *Color Atlas and Synopsis of Sexually Transmitted Diseases*, 2d ed. New York, McGraw-Hill, 2001:70–86. *A succinct, clinically oriented, extensively illustrated overview.*

Whitley RJ, Arvin AM. Herpes simplex virus infections. In: Remington JS, Klein JO, *Infectious Diseases of the Fetus and Newborn Infant*, 4th ed. Philadelphia, Saunders, 1995:354–376. *Overview of neonatal herpes.*

EPIDEMIOLOGY

Brown ZA, et al. The acquisition of herpes simplex virus during pregnancy. *N Engl J Med* 1997;337:509–515. *Prospective study showing that neonatal herpes is associated more strongly with initial than recurrent maternal herpes near term.*

Fleming DT, et al. Herpes simplex virus type 2 in the United States, 1976 to 1994. *N Engl J Med* 1997;337:1105–1111. *Report of a population-based survey showing an HSV-2-seroprevalence in adults of 22 percent, a 30 percent rise since the late 1970s.*

Schacker T, et al. Frequency of symptomatic and asymptomatic herpes simplex virus type 2 reactivations among human immunodeficiency virus-infected men. *J Infect Dis* 1998;178:1616–1622. *Demonstration of increased frequency of recurrent herpes and subclinical shedding in the presence of HIV infection.*

Wald A, et al. Reactivation of genital herpes simplex virus type 2 infection in asymptomatic seropositive persons. *N Engl J Med* 2000;342:844–850. *A study showing high rates of subclinical viral shedding in both symptomatic and asymptomatic persons with genital herpes.*

DIAGNOSIS

Ashley RL, Wald A. Genital herpes: review of the epidemic and potential use of type-specific serology. *Clin Microbiol Rev* 1999;12:1–8. *Review of type-specific serologic tests for the diagnosis of genital herpes.*

Ashley RL, et al. Premarket evaluation of the POCkit HSV-2 type-specific serologic test in culture-documented cases of genital herpes simplex virus type 2. *Sex Transm Dis* 2000;27:266–269. *Evaluation of a glycoprotein G-based type-specific serologic test; a good entrée to the literature on serologic diagnosis of HSV infection.*

DiCarlo RP, Martin DH. The clinical diagnosis of genital ulcer disease in men. *Clin Infect Dis* 1997;25:292–298. *Prospective study demonstrating that the clinical appearance of genital ulcers is insensitive and nonspecific for diagnosis.*

Koutsky L, et al. Underdiagnosis of genital herpes by current clinical and viral isolation procedures. *N Engl J Med* 1992;326:1533–1539. *Demonstration of the insensitivity of clinical assessment and viral isolation in the diagnosis of genital herpes, and the importance of type-specific serologic testing.*

Mertz KJ, et al. Etiology of genital ulcers and prevalence of human immunodeficiency virus coinfection in 10 US cities. *J Infect Dis* 1998;178:1795–1798. *A prospective study of more than 500 STD clinic patients with genital ulcer disease, showing herpes to be the predominant cause.*

TREATMENT

American College of Obstetrics and Gynecology. Management of herpes in pregnancy. *ACOG Practice Bulletin*, No. 8:1999. *Recommendations for management of herpes in pregnant women.*

Diaz-Mitoma F, et al. Oral famciclovir for the suppression of recurrent genital herpes: a randomized controlled trial. *JAMA* 1998;280:887–892. *Report of the main trial documenting efficacy and establishing recommended regimens for suppression of herpes with famciclovir.*

Patel R, et al. Impact of suppressive antiviral therapy on the health related quality of life of patients with recurrent genital herpes infection. *Sex Transm Infect*

1999;75:398–402. *Report of a multicenter trial showing that suppressive antiviral therapy improves quality of life in persons with recurrent genital herpes.*

Reitano M, et al. Valaciclovir for the suppression of recurrent genital herpes simplex virus infection: a large-scale dose range-finding study. *J Infect Dis* 1998;178: 603–610. *Results of a large, multicenter trial documenting current dosage recommendations for suppression of recurrent genital herpes with valacyclovir.*

Scott LL. Prevention of perinatal herpes: prophylactic antiviral therapy? *Clin Obstet Gynecol* 1999;42:134–148. *Review of antiviral therapy as a potential strategy to prevent neonatal herpes and herpes-related cesarean section.*

Tyring SK, et al. A randomized, placebo-controlled comparison of oral valacyclovir and acyclovir in immunocompetent patients with recurrent genital herpes infections. *Arch Dermatol* 1998;134:185–191. *Documentation of efficacy and development of recommended regimens for episodic treatment of recurrent herpes with valacyclovir.*

Wald A. New therapies and prevention strategies against genital herpes. *Clin Infect Dis* 1999; (Suppl 1):S4–S13. *A review of management strategies, prepared as background for CDC's 1998 STD treatment guidelines.*

Wald A, et al. Suppression of subclinical shedding of herpes simplex virus type 2 with acyclovir. *Ann Intern Med* 1996;124:8–15. *The first study demonstrating that antiviral therapy reduces the frequency of subclinical shedding of HSV, albeit incompletely, in women with genital herpes.*

PREVENTION AND PUBLIC HEALTH

Centers for Disease Control and Prevention. HIV prevention through early detection and treatment of sexually transmitted diseases. *Morbid Mortal Weekly Rep* 1998;46(RR-12). *Review of the influence of STDs, including genital herpes, on HIV transmission and the central role of STD control in HIV prevention.*

Corey L, et al. Recombinant glycoprotein vaccine for the prevention of genital HSV-2 infection: two randomized, double-blind placebo-controlled trials. *JAMA* 1999;282:331–340. *Report of failure of an HSV-2 vaccine candidate; an excellent entrée to the field of HSV immunization research.*

Corey L, Handsfield HH. Genital herpes and public health: addressing a global problem. *JAMA* 2000;283:791–794. *Summary of public health and prevention aspects of genital herpes.*

Fleming DT, Wasserheit JN. From epidemiological synergy to public health policy and practice: the contribution of other sexually transmitted diseases to HIV transmission. *Sex Transm Infect* 1999;75:3–17. *Overview of the influence of STDs, including herpes, on HIV transmission.*

Handsfield HH. Public health strategies to prevent genital herpes: where do we stand? *Curr Infect Dis Rep* 2000;2:25–30. *Overview of public health and prevention aspects of genital herpes.*

Stanberry LR, et al. Prospects for control of herpes simplex virus disease through immunization. *Clin Infect Dis* 2000;30:549–566. *Overview of the prospects for effective HSV vaccines and potential strategies for their use.*

INFORMATION RESOURCES FOR PERSONS WITH GENITAL HERPES OR AT RISK*

PRINT MEDIA

Ebel C. *Managing Herpes: How to Live and Love with a Chronic STD*. Research Triangle Park, NC, American Social Health Association, 1998 (238 pages). *A well-written, easy-to-read book by a leading health educator, with emphasis on the psychological and emotional aspects of genital herpes.*

Sacks SL. *The Truth About Herpes*, 5th ed. West Vancouver, Canada, Gordon Soules Book Publishers, 2001 (in press). *A comprehensive overview, with sufficiently detailed medical information to also be useful to health care providers.*

Handsfield HH. *Color Atlas and Synopsis of Sexually Transmitted Diseases*, 2d ed. New York, McGraw-Hill, 2001 (216 pages). *A succinct, extensively illustrated summary of STDs, including herpes, intended primarily for clinicians but also useful for lay persons interested in clinical and epidemiological aspects of STD.*

INTERNET WEBSITES†

Herpes Resource Center, American Social Health Association, *www.ashastd.org/hrc/index.html   ASHA is the nation's premier private, nonprofit agency devoted to prevention of STD and helping infected persons and those at risk; in addition to its excellent website, a newsletter and other printed materials are available for persons with genital herpes.*

Centers for Disease Control and Prevention, U.S. Public Health Service, *www.cdc.gov/nchstp/dstd/Genital_Herpes_facts.htm   Herpes information from the CDC, the federal government's main public health agency.*

National of Allergy and Infectious Diseases, National Institutes of Health, *www.niaid.nih.gov/factsheets/stdherp.htm   Herpes information from the NIH, the federal government's main medical research agency.*

Herpes Help, GlaxoSmithKline, Inc, *www.herpeshelp.com   Information on herpes by the producer of valacyclovir (Valtrex^R) and acyclovir (Zovirax^R), with links to other websites.*

Café Herpé, Novartis, Inc, *www.cafeherpe.com   Information on herpes, with links to other web resources, by the producer of famciclovir (Famvir^R).*

Genital Herpes, Viridae Clinical Sciences, Inc., *www.viridae.com/genital.htm   Information from a research firm that coodinates clinical trials for genital herpes and other viral infections.*

---

*Health care providers as well as patients can find useful information in the listed sources, and the American Social Health Association (319-361-8400) offers numerous patient brochures about genital herpes and other STDs, suitable for stocking in the office.

†Website addresses confirmed by the author on April 15, 2001.

National STD/AIDS Hotline, (800) 227-8922 or (800) 342-2437; Spanish language (800) 344-7432; TTY for hearing impaired (800) 243-7889. *A project of the federal Centers for Disease Control and Prevention (CDC), the Hotline is operated by the American Social Health Association; comprehensive information about all STDs, AIDS, and their prevention is available toll-free.*

National Herpes Hotline, (919) 361-8488. *Another excellent service of the American Social Health Association, for persons with herpes-related concerns that go beyond the services available at the National STD/AIDS Hotline.*

Page numbers in italics indicate figures; t *indicates table.*

Telephone resources, 38–39
Tingling sensation as prodrome, 17
Transmission of genital herpes, 4–5
Transmission of HIV, 1, 5–6
Treatment of genital herpes, 28–32
   antiviral chemotherapy for, 28–32
      in neonatal herpes, 32
      during pregnancy, 32
      principles of, 28–30, *29*
      regimens for, 30t, 30–32
   "natural" remedies for, 30
Type–specific antibody tests, 25, 26t
Tzanck test, 25

Ulcers
   facial, *19*
   labial, *16*
      in Behçet's syndrome, 28
   penile, 12, *12, 14,* 15, *15, 16,* 17
      in chancroid, 22, *22*

mimicking chancroid, 22, *23*
   vulvar, mimicking chancroid, *24*
Urethritis, 12, 13, *15,* 20
Urinary retention, 12

Vaccines, 38
Valacyclovir, 28, 30t
Varicella zoster virus, 1
Viral shedding, in subclinical
      infections, 8–9, 9t, *10*
Virologic tests, 27
Vulvar ulcers, mimicking chancroid, *24*

Websites, 38
Western blot test, 25, 26t
Women, genital herpes infection in, *16,
      17,* 20
   primary, 11–13, *14*
   recurrent, 9, *16,* 17